How to
Eat Less

**SIMPLE, PRACTICAL WAYS TO EAT LESS
WITHOUT GOING ON A DIET**

"I'm feeling so much more in control."
Barbara S

"It all makes sense. Easy to read and absorb."
Dave B

"It's fantastic. I love all the tips. A few I knew but
then as I read your explanations for each tip it
makes them seem more achievable."
Emma C

Disclaimer
Please consult your doctor before embarking on any weight
loss or exercise programmes.

This book is for people who want to achieve and maintain a
healthy weight.

ISBN: 978-1-8384948-0-3

Acknowledgements

I must give enormous thanks to my lovely client Barbara, who inspired me to write this book, and my very patient, talented and supportive husband Rick who helped me to produce it.

I would also like to take this opportunity to thank every one of my family, friends, tutors, trainers, supervisors, clients, subscribers, members and followers, who have helped me to reach this point in my life, and for encouraging me to keep going and follow my dreams.

For my Dad.

"You can't control your weight. But you CAN control your behaviour, and that affects your weight."

Claire Jones

'It is possible to fly without motors, but not without knowledge and skill.'

Wilbur Wright

About the Author Claire Jones

I'm a weight loss coach who spent 25 years 'yo-yo' dieting before finally learning to overcome my unhealthy eating behaviours. I have now maintained a healthy weight for over a decade and transformed my life. In early 2019 I left my secure employment as a senior manager in the NHS to re-train as a coach and personal trainer. I now help others to manage their weight too, by using my unique framework of developing the right mindset alongside practical knowledge and skills. My methods also support and enhance conventional weight loss approaches by helping people to choose the right one, and stick to it.

I do one-to-one and group weight loss coaching, weight loss courses, a membership subscription and run a free Facebook group. I have also written *'Preparing for Successful Weight Loss',* a manual to help those who want to lose weight to put all the right things in place for success, and help them develop their own solution, that fits with their life, their personality and their preferences.

You can find out more about my methods at
www.youronelife.co.uk

Facebook: **www.facebook.com/youronelifeuk**
Instagram: **www.instagram.com/youronelifeuk**

Preface

Thank you for purchasing my book. I decided to put it together as I have a '*Top 10 Tips to Eat Less Without Dieting'* free download which has been very popular, and I get asked to talk about it a lot. This book goes through how to apply the tips in more detail.

The idea behind these tips is that while weight loss programmes can be very effective in helping you lose weight, doing so, and keeping it off, requires a degree of commitment and dedication that isn't always sustainable, or you may not be in the right place mentally for it.

Furthermore, it can seem far more complicated than it actually is, and there are a lot of false promises made about quick fixes that claim to do the hard work for us.

Whatever route we choose, we do best when we take responsibility for our actions and understand what we are doing. We CAN be in control; when we recognise this, we hand ourselves back the power to make positive changes.

I am neither pro- nor anti-diet, as I believe that different things work for different people, but I wanted to provide an alternative, simple solution that I could share with those for whom formal dieting is not an option at the moment, for whatever reason.

In addition, it is important to be able to create sustainable habits in order to be able to keep off any weight lost in the long term.

Success lies in not just WHAT and HOW MUCH we eat, but also HOW we eat. It's also important to recognise that we can be in control of these factors, and that we have choices. If you need more help in this area, you will benefit from reading my book '*Preparing for Successful Weight Loss*' for more on developing the right mindset and learning how to develop more control over your behaviour and work out what you really want. It can be read alongside this book and will enhance your results.

I don't talk about exercise in this book because whilst it is vital for health reasons, and it is advisable to be active daily, evidence shows that it really is how much energy we consume that makes the biggest difference to our weight.

For many people, going on a diet or weight loss programme causes feelings of restriction and deprivation, and so I wanted to put something together that would help to avoid that, and to develop and maintain healthier habits, both in attitude and in practical day-to-day behaviour around food. Things that are easy to implement, apply consistently, and also improve understanding about why they are helpful. Implementing them can result in weight loss for some people without even trying to 'diet' as they help to reduce how much we eat without trying too hard or feeling so in conflict.

This handbook really focusses on the practical things we can do day-to-day to help ourselves to eat less. I consider them to be very much about developing the knowledge and particularly the skills we need to manage our weight for the long term. The more we know and understand, the better the choices we can make.

These tips are not new. I do not claim to have thought of them first. But they are what I consider to be the most helpful things that I have undertaken over the last decade that have enabled me to keep control of my behaviour around food, and therefore my weight. I talk about how I apply them.

You may already do some of them. Or they may all be new to you. But if you are already doing some of them, are you doing them consistently? I don't suggest trying to implement them all at the same time, as to do so is often not helpful - if we try to do everything at once we tend to do none of them very well. It is better to start with one or two that are either the easiest to stick to, or that will have the biggest impact, get really good at doing them consistently, and then build up from there, gradually.

So while you may already have my *Top Tips* download, I wanted to share with you in more detail how I manage them myself and give you ideas on how you might be able to apply them in your life. You can choose which ones to work on.

Do let me know how you get on with them, and which ones you find the most useful and effective. I'd love to know what you think, and I am happy to answer any questions.

Email me at **claire@youronelife.co.uk**.

Claire Jones, Founder of YourOneLife, April 2021

Contents

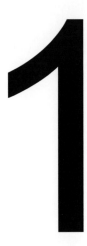

Make sure you are *physically hungry* before eating.

What does your body actually NEED?
Generally speaking, as long as we are healthy, when we are feeling physically hungry that is our body saying, 'I need food'. When we are not physically hungry, then our body doesn't usually need food. Just remembering this can help a lot.

So, this is really about paying attention to what our body needs, as opposed to what our mind wants. That's a really important distinction to make. It can be quite difficult to tell sometimes, whether we're physically hungry, or whether we're just craving something, so it's important to really listen to the signals your body is sending you.

Could you eat anything? A way to tell, if you're not sure is, to ask yourself if you could you eat anything at all, even something you don't like? Or is it just certain foods that you want to eat? If you could eat anything, then it is true physical hunger. If it's just certain things, you know it's a craving to eat something for reasons other than hunger, and it will eventually pass, whether you give in to it or not. Try drinking some water.

Use a timer. Resisting the urge to eat for reasons other than physical hunger can, of course, be quite challenging. So, if this is an issue for you, then a practical solution may be to use a timer and wait until you are actually physically hungry.

For example, if you are not feeling physically hungry, but you're having a craving, you know that eventually you WILL be physically hungry, and then you can eat whatever you are craving.

So, you're not saying *'no'*. You're just saying *'not yet'*. You can set your timer for, say, every 30 minutes, and check in with yourself to see how you're feeling, and have some distractions ready that you can do to keep your mind off it. Remember that not giving in to that craving is not going to harm you.

In my experience simply saying *'not yet'* rather than *'no'* takes a lot of the power away from the craving. You might also want to check out my blog on Emotional Eating, which will also offer some understanding about what's going on and how you can take more control. You can read it here: www.youronelife.co.uk/blog

Don't get too hungry! Be careful though. Hunger is a very powerful force and can lead to us eating too quickly when we do eat (see Tip 3), which then means we often don't control the portions (see Tip 2).

So, it's also about being aware of what is the right kind of number on the hunger scale to be eating,with 0 being full up, and 10 being

15

ravenous. 7 is generally considered to a good number to aim for. So, the best time to eat is when you're not feeling like you're starving, and so not in danger of losing control, but you're also hungry enough that your body does really need food.

You can manage this in a similar way to managing the cravings. Check in with yourself every 20-30 minutes, distract yourself in between the checks, and drink some water.

As far as the distractions go, try to choose things that you know will fully capture your attention, and, if you are not at work, are nice things to do.

Be clear in advance about the sorts of things you will choose to do... maybe read a chapter of a favourite book, watch an episode of something, do a 20-minute exercise workout, have a bath, paint your nails; something that you won't want to interrupt half-way through.

If you are at work, and in control of your workload, the same principle applies; pick a task that will take 20-30 minutes to complete.

However, if you find you are feeling continually hungry despite eating well then this is a sign that something is not quite right and needs further investigation, so do contact your doctor.

**"Thou shouldst eat to live;
not live to eat."**

Socrates

2

Use a
smaller plate
to cut down on
portion sizes.

Fool your brain! Using a smaller plate is a great way to fool your brain into thinking you're eating more than you are, especially if you combine it with Tip 3 (eating slowly). With time and practice, you will be just as satisfied.

Stay within the boundaries. I use a plate that has a ring inside it, and try to make sure that I don't go outside of the ring. Of course, it's important here not to then end up piling your plate higher to fit more food on it.

Cut down gradually. If you are used to eating much larger portions on a large plate, and piling it high, then you might need to work on this gradually.

Perhaps start with not piling it high, and then reduce the size of the plate, but you may find after a while that you wonder how you previously used to eat so much. This one in particular can make a significant difference to how much food we consume.

Portion size is one of the biggest issues my clients have, often without realising it. Thankfully it is quite easily rectified with improved awareness, and tricks like this.

**"Moderation in all things
is the best policy."**

Plautus

3

Eat slowly;

savour every mouthful.

The problem with eating too fast. When we are busy, distracted or stressed, it can be so easy to eat too fast. The problem with that is that it doesn't give our brains the chance to catch up with what and how much we're eating, so we can end up eating to fullness or beyond without realising it until it's too late. This isn't good for our waistlines or for our digestive health.

The accepted advice to eat more slowly is to eat without distractions, to chew our food a certain number of times before swallowing it, and to not load the fork or spoon up until we've finished the last mouthful.

Now, while chewing our food properly and not loading the fork up too soon are certainly good advice which I would absolutely encourage you to follow, personally I have never found it particularly helpful to eat without any distractions at all.

So, I am going to be a little controversial here...

Eating with or without distractions? When I concentrate fully on the food I'm eating, without distractions, I really don't like it. In fact, I find I end up eating faster because I want to get it over with!

So, I actually find it slows me down MORE to havesome kind of distraction when I am eating, such as using the internet.

Actually, when we think about it, this isn't really much different to having conversation at the dinner table, as we eat, which naturally slows us down.

In modern society many of us tend to do less of that, and more people eat in front of the TV without conversation these days, so eating CAN become mindless, and it's way too easy then to eat too fast.

However, I find that by catching up on social media, for example, while eating my meals, I naturally eat more slowly as I put my cutlery down in between mouthfuls. I also use my hands to scroll, or type, and I do make sure I pay some attention to what I am eating as well, and I enjoy it.

Note: this is only if I am eating alone. I would find it rude to do this in company... in which case the conversation would be the distraction.

I am not suggesting that this is what you should do but it does work for me. You will need to experiment to see what works for you.

I find that, combined with controlling portion size, and only eating when hungry, this is very effective for me.

The only the only time I find that it doesn't work so well is if I suddenly get stressed by something that I have read or seen, but being aware of this helps me to watch out for it.

Challenge yourself. Time how long it currently takes you to eat your main meals. Then challenge yourself to make it last a little bit longer each time, until you feel you have got it right.

Use a teaspoon. Another little tip that goes nicely with this is to use a teaspoon in place of a dessert spoon. This works well for breakfast cereals and desserts, and really helps to slow me down.

"The two most powerful warriors are patience and time."

Leo Tolstoy

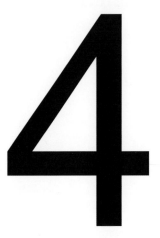

Stop eating when you are satisfied, and *before you get full*.

Put less food on your plate. Many people find stopping eating when they still have food on their plate one of the hardest things to do, especially if what they are eating is particularly tasty.

So, the best way to manage this, is to work on Tip2 (using a smaller plate).

If you are getting full, but you can't stop eating, then that's a sign to tell you that you need to put less on your plate next time, and/or to cook less. Really pay attention to this as it is excellent feedback to guide your future behaviour.

Wait 20 minutes. So, if you have got to the end of your meal, and you're tempted to go back for seconds, that's when the 20-minute rule is really important, as research has shown that's how long it takes for the brain to recognise we have had enough to eat.

So, quite simply, wait 20 minutes before going back. If after 20 minutes you still want more and you feel you are definitely still physically hungry, then by all means have more. But if not, then don't.

Use distractions. You can use the distractions mentioned in Tip 1, and then check in with yourself after 20 minutes. Chances are you will feel very differently - and if you don't, then see if you can work out whether you really are still hungry, or just want more food.

Have a cup of tea. One thing I find helpful is to have a cup of tea after a meal. By the time I have finished it I really don't feel like I want any more food. It doesn't have to be tea, but a drink of some kind that is low in calories can really help.

Leave something on your plate. Another thing you can try is to get into the habit of always leaving something on your plate, even if it's only one mouthful to begin with. That way, you can build your skills of self-control in stopping eating when you are satisfied, and break that tendency always to have to finish what's on your plate. You don't. Tune in to what your body is telling you.

Don't worry. If you are worried about feeling hungry again soon, that's ok, as if you really are hungry, you can eat!

If not, and it's a craving, then you need to manage it in the ways described in Tip 1. However, as previously mentioned, if you find you are feeling continually hungry despite eating well then this is a sign that something is not quite right and needs further investigation, so do contact your doctor.

5

Dispose of any leftovers on your plate or in the kitchen *immediately*.

You are not a human dustbin. It's all too easy to pick at food if we leave leftovers lying around, either on our plate, someone else's plate, or in the kitchen.

So, in order to avoid this, it is wise to get rid of them as soon as possible, either by refrigerating or freezing them, or putting them in the food waste. It really isn't a waste if they're not going on YOUR waist! Remove them from your sight and from temptation immediately.

Sunk costs. There is a term called 'sunk costs' which I find helpful to use in this scenario. It refers to money that has already been spent and which cannot be recovered.

We can apply it quite easily to food as well. Once we've cooked or bought a meal, it is no longer possible to recover the cost, whether we eat it or not. It is a sunk cost.

Eating it yourself when you are not hungry will do you no favours at all, and will only add inches to your waistline and all the other associated problems with that. So just get rid of it, and cook less next time.

Put barriers in the way. Make sure that any temptations are kept out of sight, so that you cannot just grab at them mindlessly when you walk past.

The more barriers you can put in the way of being able to eat something, the less likely you are to eat something opportunistically.

For example, putting the leftovers in a container with a lid on it, at the back of the fridge means that you will have to go through several steps to actually get to the food, which will give you more of a chance to remind yourself of what you really want, and change your course of action.

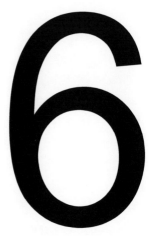

Avoid processed foods wherever possible.

What's wrong with processed foods? When we eat heavily processed foods, which tend to be higher in refined sugar, our bodies digest them quickly and easily and we crave more of them ... making it so much harder to maintain our resolve. They are also thought to be linked to various health problems. You wouldn't put low quality fuel into a high-performance sports car and then expect it to work properly, so think of your body in the same way.

We also don't get much 'bang for our buck' - they are often very calorie dense, while being light on nutrition. The body digests them really quickly so we don't stay full for long and can quickly feel hungry or have cravings again soon after.

Furthermore, the more sugary things we consume, the more we WANT to consume, yet giving in to the cravings for them does not solve the problem, it only provides temporary relief.

None of this does any good for our confidence in our ability to lose weight, especially as a lot of processed foods are also very high in fat, and therefore calories; much more than we may realise.

What to have instead. I like to think about eating what we are *designed* to eat. We are not designed to eat heavily processed foods, but we ARE designed to eat a wide range of foods that are in as natural a state as possible (but properly cooked and washed of course). Some of these foods, such as broccoli, lettuce, and strawberries are so low in calories that we can have very generous amounts of them, which helps to keep us satisfied.

Much research shows that choosing minimally processed food may help with things like hormonal imbalances, insulin resistance, intolerances, energy levels and sleep quality, and can make us feel so much healthier on a day-to-day basis.

It is possible to eat minimally processed foods on a low budget, and can also be extremely enjoyable if we take the time to learn how to cook lower calorie healthy meals. With a bit of effort and imagination it is very possible to eat really healthily and enjoy it. It's not all cottage cheese and celery!

So always aim to choose foods that are as close to their natural state as possible, and avoid adding extra sugar. E.g., you could have rolled porridge oats with some dried fruit rather than adding sugar or syrup to sweeten it. Frozen and tinned foods are fine if they are still in their original form as they retain their nutrients just as well if not better than fresh foods that are several days old. They are also often cheaper. Just make sure the tins of fruit, for example, use water or natural juices and not syrup.

A quick search on Google or Pinterest will give you lots of ideas or you can check out my blog articles for more information.
www.youronelife.co.uk/blog

Of course, it's nice to have *some* processed foods because they are very enjoyable and won't do too much harm for most of us in moderation as long as we are in good health and the majority of our diet is of good quality and minimally processed.

So, by all means have some treats but make sure they are limited (see Tip 7).

Check out the NHS Eatwell website for more information about all the different varieties of unprocessed foods you can eat. The NHS Eatwell Guide gives a good visual representation of how much they should feature in our daily or weekly intake. See page 67 for the link as well as links to other websites that can help you with making better food choices, including interesting and tasty recipes.

"Let food be thy medicine and medicine be thy food."

Hippocrates

7

Have some treats to look forward to but *put some limits on them*.

The 80/20 principle. For most of us who struggle with our weight, it's not realistic to cut out treats altogether, nor do we want to, so we have to find a way to manage them.

I like to use the 80/20 principle where roughly 80% of my food is good quality, minimally processed, lighter on calories, but dense on nutrition, and then I've got 20% to play with.

This doesn't mean I will have an unlimited quantity of treats. It just means that for the remaining 20% of my calories, it doesn't matter if they are not so nutritious.

Most days I will have a treat of some kind of processed food but the vast majority of my intake is healthy. I make compromises with myself on a daily basis.

For example, if I want to have more of one thing, it might mean having less of something else. I advise people who are trying to lose weight, however, to aim for a 90/10 split, rather than 80/20, but there's always room for a bit of indulgence, as trying to cut them out for many people is not realistic or sustainable.

Just be mindful that eating sweet things can make you want to eat *more* sweet things, so cutting them out for a while might be worthwhile, in order to break the cycle.

You don't have to have your dessert straight away. One of the things that is very common is feeling the need to have a dessert after a meal.

The problem with this is that it often means continuing to eat when we're no longer hungry. A way that I manage this is to wait until later, and then have my dessert. Or, if I am eating out, I will have a little of it and then ask the restaurant to box up the rest so I can have it later when I am feeling hungry. I find doing this means I enjoy it so much more and I don't end up feeling unpleasantly full.

You don't have to have a dessert at all! Getting in the habit of saying no sometimes is a good thing. Maybe think about limiting desserts to certain days or meals rather than every day or meal, if you are in the habit of having them all the time. Remember, habits can be broken!

Smaller portions, and less often, but be careful of bite-sized treats. Many manufacturers now offer smaller alternatives, which is great in theory, but we can often end up eating more than if we had the usual size because we underestimate how many calories they have, and end up having too many.

So, it's important to know and understand what's in them, decide how many to have beforehand, stickto the decision, and put the packet away.

Also consider how many times you are having treats, and see if you can cut this down.

Lower calorie alternatives. There are lots of swaps you can make to really cut down on calories... lower fat cream, sugar-free jelly, mini-lollies, fresh fruit salad instead of trifle, yogurt instead of ice cream .... etc.

We can make lower calorie foods very interesting and enjoyable with a bit of imagination. See the links on page 67 for recipe ideas.

"Moderation tends to increase enjoyment and makes pleasure even greater."

Democritus

8

Understand how much you are eating by using a tracker.

Do you know how much you are spending? I like to manage my food and drink intake in a similar way to how I manage my money, and be fully aware that it's all too easy to go on a spending spree!

Imagine going to a shopping centre or shopping online .... spending £20 in Marks and Spencer, £14.99 in Boots...£3.50 in WH Smith...£18 in Next...£15 in the Body Shop...£8.99 in Costa, and £20 in Primark.

Unless you were using cash and could see it disappearing, or were using a spending app that tots it up as you go, would you have realised that you had spent over £100 until you got home and added it all up? Or til your bank statement arrived... if you check it at all....

It's the same when we eat throughout the day. Each meal or snack on its own may not be very high in calories, but when we add them all up, they can end up taking us over what we need each day and as a result we will put on weight.

How to find out. As a first step, I always advise anyone who doesn't understand why they are not losing weight, or why they are putting it on, to spend a week or two weighing and tracking their food and drink using an app that will record their calorie intake.

It is time very well spent as it is a really good way to educate ourselves about what and how much we are eating, and help us to make better decisions. It's important to do it in real time though, not later, as it's so easy to forget what we've had.

It's like shopping with cash. You can see how much you're spending and how much you've got left, and once it's gone it's gone.

The importance of accuracy. It is vital to be accurate though, as the data is only as accurate as what is entered. That means weighing and measuring and not guessing, and paying attention to ensure the correct quantities are chosen.

Isn't that too much effort? In my opinion, no. Weighing, measuring and tracking will really help you to understand more about your body, your food and your exercise choices.

It will also enable you to make much better decisions on a day-to-day basis, and stop laying excuses at the door of medication, hormones, menopause etc. and going down the road of spending money on things that promise to, but don't actually, solve the problem.

It's not too hard, or boring, if you do it properly. There are lots of apps and websites that help to make it as easy as possible, such as `www.myfitnesspal.com`, and it can be really interesting, eye-opening, and most of all empowering since it can enable you to take better control. It's an extremely worthwhile exercise.

You don't need to do it forever; only until you've got a handle on things.

However, it's good to go back to if you stop getting results.

I still track from time to time. It's the first thing I do if I feel things are slipping.

It gives me full awareness and enables me to nip any problems in the bud.

The time that it's most important to do it is the time that we least want to – when we've overeaten. But the sooner we face up to what we're doing, the sooner we take back control and limit any damage. I no longer allow myself to bury my head in the sand. For more on this read my *'Preparing for Successful Weight Loss'* book.

"Nothing in life is to be feared. It is only to be understood."

Marie Curie

9

Pay close attention to how many calories you are drinking - *they count too*.

What's wrong with drinks? It's so easy to drink many of our calories. If you are used to having 5 or 6 cups of tea or coffee with milk each day, you will be having up to 200 calories.

If you have 2 sugars in each of them that's another 160-200 calories, so you could be having 400 calories just from tea and coffee alone.

Then if you are drinking any juices, or milkshakes, or lattes, cappuccinos, hot chocolate or anything alcoholic, you'll be adding a few hundred more.

The UK government guidelines state women need 2000 calories and men need 2500 a day to maintain weight, so a significant proportion of our daily intake could be coming from our drinks before we've counted any food!

Still wondering why you can't lose weight?

What to do instead. Try to get in the habit of drinking more water - not only is it absolutely ideal for the body, for so many reasons, including helping the body burn fat and get rid of waste products, it will also help you to manage hunger and sugar cravings.

There's no need to avoid tea, coffee and other drinks. Just be mindful of how many you are having, and put some limits on them.

A few words about alcohol. Not only does alcohol contain a significant number of calories, it also lowers our resolve, can stimulate our appetite and can impact on our sleep quality and hormones, which can then also stimulate our appetite the following day.

So, if we are drinking in the evening, we're more likely to resort to late night snacking, and of the processed variety, or fatty takeaways. We may also end up eating more food the following day.

Furthermore, the body will process the alcohol first, meaning much of the food you eat is not needed for energy and will be more likely to be stored as fat.

So, with this in mind, it's a good idea to have a very clear plan of how to manage your alcohol and food intake BEFORE you start drinking if you don't want it to derail you. Think of all the likely obstacles and write down your plan of how you will deal with them so that you can set your intentions firmly in advance.

10

Have healthy, *low calorie snacks available.*

Choose things you really like. It doesn't have to be cottage cheese and celery, if that's not your thing. But it's important to have healthy, tasty snacks available that you like, as it will stop you from getting too hungry and losing control, and choosing less healthy alternatives.

Ensuring they contain some protein is important as this will help keep you satisfied until you are ready for your next main meal. It will also help to preserve your lean tissue (e.g., your muscles and organs) and therefore your metabolism, so that you are more likely to keep your lost weight off.

My favourite go-to snack when at home is authentic Greek yogurt with strawberries, and a tiny sprinkling of crunchy granola.

There are lots of ideas on Google and Pinterest if you search for healthy low-calorie snacks.

Just be careful to measure the quantities and adjust if need be.

Don't eat them just because they are there. It is important, though, to follow the principles in Tip 1, and make sure you are physically hungry. Don't use it as an excuse to eat, just because they are there. Avoiding sugary snacks will really help.

Keep them in places you will need them. I always have a couple of snacks in my handbag and in my car, so that if I get caught out unexpectedly and start to feel hungry, I have things to fall back on and therefore avoid the temptations that might otherwise lead me astray when out and about.

But be careful of packaged snacks. Some packaged snacks, whilst labelled as healthy, can be very high in various different types of sugar and it can be all too easy to eat more than one of them.

So, try to follow the principles of sticking to as unprocessed and natural a snack as possible, and check the labels.

Watch out for flapjacks; they are packed with sugar and fat, and therefore extremely high in calories.

Check out the link on page 67 for a very helpful article from the British Heart Foundation about understanding food labels, to help you with what to look for.

Summary

1

Pay attention to your body. Make sure you are physically hungry (but don't wait til you're 'starving') before eating.

2

Use a small plate to cut down on portion sizes.

3

Eat slowly; savour every mouthful.

4

Stop eating when you are satisfied, and BEFORE you get full. If you're not sure, wait 20 minutes.

5

Dispose of any leftovers on your plate or in the kitchen immediately. It is NOT a waste if it means they are not going on YOUR WAIST!

6

Avoid processed food wherever possible.

7

Have some treats to look forward to, but put some limits on them, eg smaller treats, better alternatives, and/or less often.

8

Understand how much you are eating by using a tracker but make sure you enter the right information!

9

Pay attention to how many calories you are drinking - they count too! Drink water instead.

10

Have healthy, low calorie snacks available at all times to help you avoid or manage temptations and tide you over to stop you getting TOO hungry and risk losing control.

Remember, these tips only work if we actually DO them, and do them consistently. So now it's over to you!

Bonus Tips

If you have trouble with snacking and portion control, I am confident that applying at least some of the tips in this book will help you to get on top of your eating behaviours too. But if you need more help, you might want to check out these bonus tips from my book *'Preparing for Successful Weight Loss'* which you can buy on my website.

Losing weight is hard for many people because ultimately, we want two different things at the same time; to eat as much as we want, and to be a healthy weight, and everything that means to us. So, we are in constant conflict. In my opinion itis vital to continually work on our mindset alongside our practical efforts, so that over time we **change what we want, and the process becomes easier,** not just to lose weight, but to keep it off.

These bonus tips help people to do just that.

Cultivate your environment
Think about what and who is around you. Is it supportive? Remove as much as possible that is unhelpful, and add in as much as you can that will

help you. Link up with other people who are trying to do the same, and support each other.

Be clear what you want and set realistic goals
Have a clear vision of what you want to achieve and spend time every day reminding yourself of it. This will really help you to make better decisions when faced with temptation. Make sure it's achievable though, and set realistic, not idealistic goals! Progress is far more important than perfection.

Develop some affirmations
Work on things you can say to yourself daily that you can use when you are tempted, that can instantly bring you back to your goals so you can make the right decisions.

Look how far you've come
Take time regularly to recognise what you've achieved, not just with weight loss, but other things as well. Remind yourself of all the incredible things you're capable of.

Take it one day at a time
Treat each day like a mini-goal and focus your efforts on making it the best it can be, and don't worry about tomorrow. If you do this, the results will naturally follow.

A success story

My husband lost over 4 stone using some of the tips in this book.

He had gained weight slowly over a number of years as a result of developing some less-than-healthy habits including mindless snacking and excessive portion sizes.

He lost 4 and a half stone by following some of the tips that I describe in this book and has now successfully maintained his loss for over 6 months by continuing to follow them, and without any effort.

He has not followed a 'diet' and has transformed his eating behaviours. I am incredibly proud of him, and very relieved as he had been suffering some weight-related health problems which appear to have been fully resolved so far.

You can read more about him on my website.
www.youronelife.co.uk

"These techniques not only worked to help me lose weight, but they continue to work to help me keep it off. Best of all, none of it is exactly difficult to stick to."
Rick Jones

Further reading and resources

Visit my website
Have a look at my website for more information about how I work, and for my other books and resources, including tasty, filling recipes.
www.youronelife.co.uk

Healthy Eating Advice and Ideas
Visit the NHS Eat Well Guide:
www.nhs.uk/live-well/eat-well/the-eatwell-guide
for healthy eating advice. The NHS also have a free NHS 12-week weight loss plan that is worth checking out.

Visit the Precision Nutrition website
www.precisionnutrition.com/blog
for advice on healthy eating habits. This link is particularly helpful if you don't want to count calories.
www.precisionnutrition.com/what-should-i-eat-infographic

Take a look at this British Heart Foundation article on Understanding Food Labels.
www.bhf.org.uk/informationsupport/support/healthy-living/healthy-eating/food-labelling

Visit Pinch of Nom www.pinchofnom.com

for lots of tasty, nutritious lower calorie recipe ideas.

Help with tracking and identifying where extra calories are coming from

Try MyFitnessPal www.myfitnesspal.com for tracking your food and drink. There is a premium version but the free version is enough for many people's needs.

Take a look at the Secret Eaters TV programme which demonstrates how easy it is to overeat without realising it. It isn't broadcast anymore but you can find episodes by searching on Google or YouTube.

YOU ONLY GET
ONE LIFE

Let me help you make the best of it

Printed in Great Britain
by Amazon